SIRTF
DIET
COOKBOOK

New Sirtfood Diet Recipes to Help You Lose Weight and Improve your Lifestyle

Shannen Gallowey

© Copyright 2021 by - Shannen Gallowey - All rights reserved.

The following Book is reproduced below with the goal of providing information that is as accurate and reliable as possible. Regardless, purchasing this Book can be seen as consent to the fact that both the publisher and the author of this book are in no way experts on the topics discussed within and that any recommendations or suggestions that are made herein are for entertainment purposes only. Professionals should be consulted as needed prior to undertaking any of the action endorsed herein.

This declaration is deemed fair and valid by both the American Bar Association and the Committee of Publishers Association and is legally binding throughout the United States.

Furthermore, the transmission, duplication, or reproduction of any of the following work including specific information will be considered an illegal act irrespective of if it is done electronically or in print. This extends to creating a secondary or tertiary copy of the work or a recorded copy and is only allowed with the express written consent from the Publisher. All additional right reserved.

The information in the following pages is broadly considered a truthful and accurate account of facts and as such, any inattention, use, or misuse of the information in question by the reader will render any resulting actions solely under their purview. There are no scenarios in which the publisher or the original author of this work can be in any fashion deemed liable for any hardship or damages that may befall them after undertaking information described herein.

Additionally, the information in the following pages is intended only for informational purposes and should thus be thought of as universal. As befitting its nature, it is presented without assurance regarding its prolonged validity or interim quality. Trademarks that are mentioned are done without written consent and can in no way be considered an endorsement from the trademark holder.

TABLE OF CONTENTS

Introduction 7
Sirtfood Recipes 11
    Vegetable Smoothie 12
    Smoked Salmon Omelet 13
    Sirt Fruit Salad 14
    Banana Blueberry Pancakes with Apple Compote 15
    Raw Buckwheat Breakfast Porridge 17
    Sirtfood Green Juice 18
    Three-Pepper Breakfast Burritos 19
    Pomegranate and Cranberry Smoothie 20
    Carrots and Cauliflower Spread 22
    Sirt Muesli 23
    Apple and Pecan Bowls 24
    Spicy Lentils Vegetable Soup 25
    Cauliflower Curry 26
    Strawberry & Citrus Blend 28
    Raspberry and Blackcurrant Jelly 29
    Mince Stuffed Eggplants 30
    Turkey Curry 31
    Turkey Escalope with Sage, Trick and Parsley and Spiced Cauliflower 'Couscous' 32
    Baked Cod with Kale, Chicory and White Beans 34
    Chicken Fajitas 36

Green Tea Smoothie 37

Turmeric Couscous with Edamame Beans 38

Crude Brownie Bites 39

Sirtfood Pizza 40

Beef Burger with Sweet Potato Fries 42

Yellow Lentil Soup with Chilli, Ginger and Turmeric................ 44

Turmeric Tea... 46

Potato Salad 47

Black Bean Salsa 49

Kale and Butternut Bowls 50

Sweet Potato Soup 52

Easy Shrimp Salad 54

New Saag Paneer 55

Corn Spread 57

Moroccan Leeks Snack.. 58

Best Ever Bran Muffins 59

Stew with Green Vegetables... 61

Tuscan Bean Stew... 63

Chicken Breakfast Skillet.. 65

Green Shakshuka 66

Buckwheat Superfood Muesli 68

Pineapple & Cucumber Smoothie 69

Roasted Cajun Nuts 70

Frozen Chocolate Grapes.. 71

Choc Chip Granola 73

Walnut Butter... 75

Chocolate Dessert with Dates and Walnuts.............................. 76

Blueberry Smoothie 77

Avocado, Celery & Pineapple Smoothie..................................... 78

Sirtfood Bites 79

Introduction

Sirtfood - the new trend diet.

In the United Kingdom, two celebrity nutritionists collaborating with a health club founded The Sirtfood Diet. They market the diet as a ground-breaking modern health and wellbeing strategy that works by turning on the "skinny gene," This diet focuses on Sirtuin (SIRT) research, a group of seven body proteins that have been shown to regulate numerous roles, inflammation, including metabolism and lifespan. Certain organic plant compounds can increase the number of such proteins, and diets containing them have been called 'Sirtfoods.'

The Sirtfood Diet's listing of the "Top 20 Sirtfoods" includes:

- Extra-virgin Olive Oil
- Dark Chocolate (85% Cocoa) Matcha Green Tea Buckwheat
- Turmeric Walnuts
- Arugula (Rocket) Bird's Eye Chili Lovage
- Kale
- Red Wine Strawberries Onions
- Soy Parsley
- Medjool Dates Red Chicory Blueberries Capers
- Coffee

In the diet, Sirtfoods and calorie restriction are mixed, enabling the body to produce greater amounts of Sirtuins.

The diet creators suggest it will result in dramatic weight loss by following the Sirtfood Diet while maintaining muscle mass and protecting you from chronic disease. After completing the diet, all are allowed to start adding sirtfoods and the diet's signature green juice into their regular diet.

Advantages and disadvantages of the Sirtfood Diet

As with any other diet, the Sirtfood Diet has advantages and disadvantages.

Advantages:

Sirtuin-containing foods can have a positive influence on the metabolism and help to change quickly. There is initially a large amount of water excreted, which leads to relatively rapid weight loss. Consequences of the increased metabolism are a conversion of the fat cells and increased excretion. The organism is fundamentally detoxified and the bodyweight decreases as a result. An improved metabolism leads to an optimized immune system, which leads to improved protection against tumor formation and other diseases. It is assumed that the optimized metabolism can extend life by several years.

In addition to the positive metabolic processes, the sirtuin-containing products support muscle building, as already mentioned at the beginning. Thus, in addition to losing weight or maintaining the weight, intensive physical training can also be carried out. Strictly speaking, there are no foods on the sirtfood diet that are specifically prohibited. Of course, sirtuin-rich foods are to be preferred, but other products may also be consumed from time to time and in small quantities.

Although a maximum daily amount of calories is provided, you don't need to worry about feeling hungry. All dishes that can be created with these foods are wonderfully full and with a good eating plan, you can easily stick to the diet.

During the sirtfood diet, stored fat, called white fat, melts. The storage fat is replaced by the brown fat, but this fat is an energy eater, which therefore contributes to the weight loss effect.

Disadvantage:

Most diets have already been tested for their effectiveness by renowned scientists. One can rely on their statements and results. In the case of the sirtfood diet, these results are still pending, as there have only been small studies so far and these have not yet provided any conclusive evidence that corresponds to scientific standards.

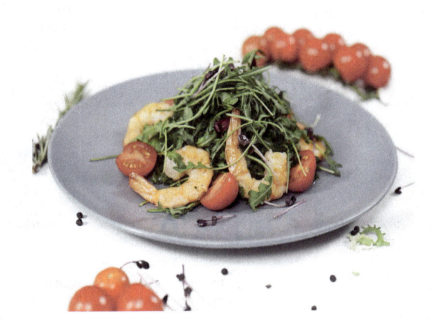

Sirtfood Recipes

Vegetable Smoothie

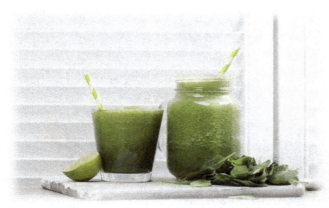

Time required: 10 minutes

Servings: 02

INGREDIENTS

75 g green cabbage
30 g rocket
5 g parsley
2-3 stalks of celery
½ green apple
1 teaspoon lemon juice
1 teaspoon matcha tea

STEPS FOR COOKING

1. Mix all ingredients, except for matcha tea, together until the desired consistency is achieved.
2. Before serving, add 1 teaspoon of matcha tea and stir.

Smoked Salmon Omelet

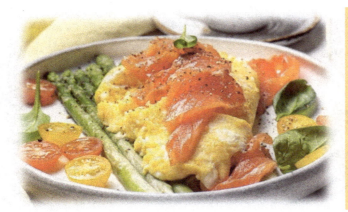

Time required: 10 minutes

Servings: 01

INGREDIENTS

2 medium-size eggs
3½ ounces sliced smoked salmon
½ tsp capers
½ tbsp rocket (chopped)
1 tsp fresh parsley (chopped)
1 tsp extra-virgin olive oil

STEPS FOR COOKING

1. In a bowl, whisk the eggs.
2. To the eggs, add the smoked salmon, capers, rocket, and parsley. In a frying pan, heat the oil until hot but not smoking.
3. Add the egg mixture to the pan, and with a spatula, move the mixture around the frying pan until it is even.
4. Turn down the heat, and allow the omelet to cook through.
5. Slide the spatula around the edges of the pan, and fold the omelet in half. Serve and enjoy.

Sirt Fruit Salad

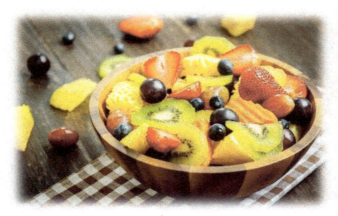

Time required: 15 minutes

Servings: 01

INGREDIENTS

½ cup newly made green tea
1 tsp nectar
1 orange, split
1 apple, cored and generally hacked
10 red seedless grapes
10 blueberries

STEPS FOR COOKING

1. Stir the nectar into a large portion of some green tea. At the point when disintegrated, add the juice of a large portion of the orange.
2. Leave to cool.
3. Chop the other portion of the orange and spot in a bowl along with the hacked apple, grapes and blueberries.
4. Pour over the cooled tea and leave to soak for a couple of moments prior to serving.

Banana Blueberry Pancakes with Apple Compote

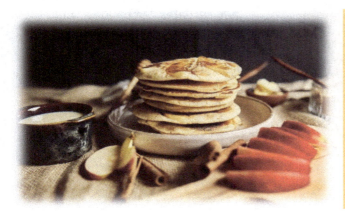

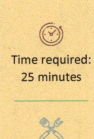

Time required: 25 minutes

Servings: 04

INGREDIENTS

Pancakes:
5 ounces rolled oats
6 bananas (peeled)
6 eggs
2 tsp baking powder
¼ tsp salt
8 ounces blueberries
Butter (as needed)

Compote:
2 apples (cored and coarsely chopped)
5 dates (pitted)
1 tbsp freshly squeezed lemon juice
¼ tsp cinnamon powder
2 tbsp water
Pinch of salt

STEPS FOR COOKING

1. First, prepare the pancakes. In a dry high-speed food blender, pulse the oats for 60 seconds to create oat flour.
2. Add the bananas to the blender, followed by the eggs, baking powder, and salt. Pulse the mixture to create a smooth batter for 2 minutes.
3. Transfer the batter to a bowl, and fold in the berries. Set aside to rest for 10 minutes while the baking powder activates.
4. Add a dollop of butter to a frying pan set over moderate to high heat. Add 2-3 spoonfuls of the pancake mix to the pan and fry until the bottom is golden. Flip the pancake over and cook on the reverse side.

INGREDIENTS	STEPS FOR COOKING
	5. **For the Compote:** Add the ingredients (apples, dates, lemon juice, and cinnamon powder) to a food processor. Add 2 tablespoons of water along with a pinch of salt. On the pulse setting process to create a chunky consistency compote. 6. Serve the pancakes with the compote and enjoy.

Raw Buckwheat Breakfast Porridge

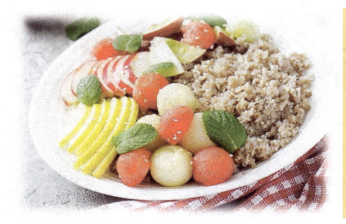

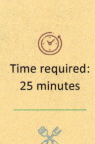

Time required: 25 minutes

Servings: 04

INGREDIENTS

2 cups raw groats of buckwheat, soaked overnight, rinsed and drained
1 cup almond milk
Quarter cup maple syrup
1 teaspoon cinnamon
1 teaspoon vanilla extract, or 1 vanilla bean, seeds scooped out
1 tablespoon of crushed flax meal
1 pinch sea salt
1/3 cup shredded, unsweetened coconut

STEPS FOR COOKING

1. In the food processor, put the buckwheat groats & pulse few times to breakdown.
2. Maple syrup, Almond milk, vanilla bean, cinnamon, sea salt, and flax are applied and refined until the mixture is smooth (but with some residual texture).
3. Pulse and change the seasonings in the cocoon. Divide the porridge into four bowls and serve with chopped almonds, fresh berries, or sliced bananas.

SHANNEN GALLOWEY
Sirtfood Diet Cookbook

Sirtfood Green Juice

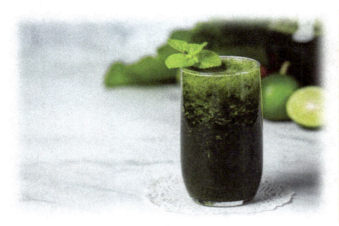

Time required: 15 minutes

Servings: 01

INGREDIENTS

1 tbsp. parsley
1 stalk celery
1 apple
½ lemon
1 cucumber
1 stalk celery
1 apple
3 mint leaves

STEPS FOR COOKING

1. Choose one of the recipes above.
2. Add all ingredients into a juicer and extract the juice according to the manufacturer's method.
3. In case you don't have one, add all the ingredients to a blender and pulse until well combined.
4. Filter the juice through a fine-mesh strainer and transfer it into a glass. Top with water if needed. Serve immediately.

Three-Pepper Breakfast Burritos

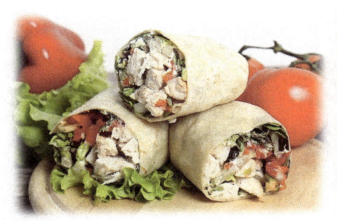

Time required: 25 minutes

Servings: 04

INGREDIENTS

1/4 cup sliced green onions
1/2 medium green bell pepper, chopped
1/2 medium red bell pepper, chopped
1/2 medium yellow bell pepper, chopped
6 eggs
2 tablespoons milk
1/2 teaspoon salt
1/8 teaspoon pepper
4 (7 or 8-inch) flour tortillas, heated
2 oz. (1/2 cup) shredded hot pepper Monterey Jack cheese

STEPS FOR COOKING

1. Melt the margarine over the moderate flame in a medium, nonstick skillet.
2. Add bell peppers and onions; cook 2 to 3 minutes or until veggies are tender and crisp, simmer gently. In the meantime, combine the eggs, milk, salt and pepper in a medium bowl; whisk well. In a skillet, pour the egg mixture over the vegetables. Bring to a simmer; cook until eggs are set but still moist, stirring frequently, or 4 to 6 minutes.
3. Spoon egg mixture on warm tortillas for serving; sprinkle with cheese.
4. Roll up.

Pomegranate and Cranberry Smoothie

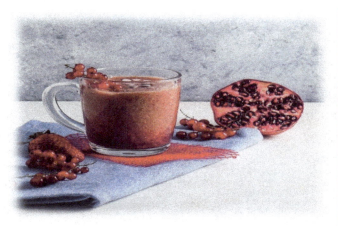

Time required: 15 minutes

Servings: 02

INGREDIENTS

1 pomegranate
100 g fresh cranberries, alternatively the juice
150 g natural yogurt
250 ml milk Ice cubes liquid sweetener as desired

STEPS FOR COOKING

1. Cut out a small piece from the stalk of the pomegranate. Then carefully break the fruit into two parts over a bowl with a little pressure so that most of the stones fall out of the shell. If necessary, work the pomegranate with thin rubber or disposable gloves, as the juice is very colored.
2. Set aside about 1 tbsp of the pomegranate seeds. Pour the rest of the cranberries and yoghurt into a suitable mixing vessel and puree with a hand blender.
3. Sweeten with a little sweetener to your own taste, stir in the milk and ice cubes and mix in again briefly with the hand blender.

INGREDIENTS	STEPS FOR COOKING
	4. Divide between 2 glasses and serve garnished with the remaining pomegranate seeds.

Carrots and Cauliflower Spread

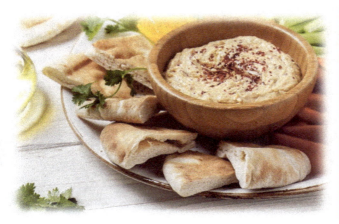

Time required: 55 minutes

Servings: 04

INGREDIENTS

1 c. carrots, sliced
2 c. cauliflower florets
½ c. cashews
2 ½ c. water
1 c. almond milk
1 tsp. garlic powder
¼ tsp. smoked paprika

STEPS FOR COOKING

1. Mix the carrots with the cauliflower, the cashews and the water in a small pot, stir, cover, bring to a boil over medium heat, simmer for 40 minutes, rinse and mix.
2. Apply the almond milk, garlic and paprika powder, pulse well, cut into small bowls and eat well.
3. Enjoy!

Sirt Muesli

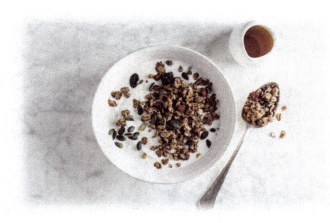

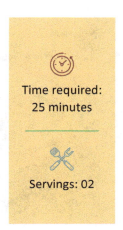

Time required: 25 minutes

Servings: 02

INGREDIENTS

0.7 oz. buckwheat chips
0.35 oz. buckwheat puffs
0.5 oz. coconut chips or parched coconut
1.5 oz. Medjool dates, hollowed and slashed
0.5 oz. pecans, cleaved
0.35 oz. cocoa nibs
3.5 oz. strawberries, hulled and cleaved
3.5 oz. plain Greek yogurt (or veggie lover elective, for example, soya or coconut yogurt)

STEPS FOR COOKING

1. Blend the entirety of the above ingredients together, possibly adding the yogurt and strawberries prior to serving in the event that you are making it in mass.

Apple and Pecan Bowls

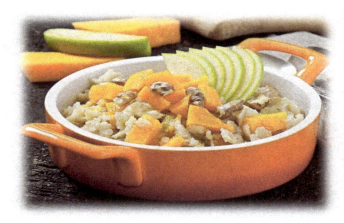

Time required: 25 minutes

Servings: 04

INGREDIENTS

4 big apples, cored, peeled and cubed
2 teaspoons lemon juice
¼ cup pecans, chopped

STEPS FOR COOKING

1. In a bowl, mix apples with lemon juice, and pecans and toss.
2. Divide into small bowls and serve as a snack.

Spicy Lentils Vegetable Soup

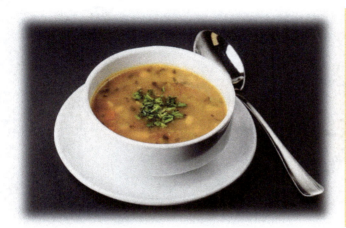

Time required: 35 minutes

Servings: 01

INGREDIENTS

1 teaspoon extra-virgin olive oil plus
30 g red onion
30 g celery
30 g carrot
1 Birds Eye Chili
1 clove of garlic
1 teaspoon ground turmeric
1 tsp curry powder
500 ml vegetable broth
50 g red lentils
1 teaspoon chopped parsley

STEPS FOR COOKING

1. Heat the olive oil over low to moderate temperature in a small saucepan and fry the onion, celery and carrot for 2-3 minutes, until soft.
2. Garnish with chili, garlic and spices and simmer for another minute. Connect the lentils and vegetable stock and get it to a boil.
3. For 30 minutes, cook gently and stir from time to time so that nothing sticks to the floor. Stir in the parsley and serve with a splash of extra virgin olive oil after the lentils have broken down, and they have excellent soupy consistency.

Cauliflower Curry

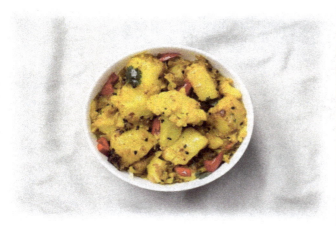

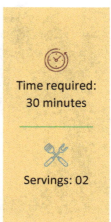

Time required: 30 minutes

Servings: 02

INGREDIENTS

½ teaspoon ground cumin
½ teaspoon ground coriander
½ teaspoon ground turmeric
1 teaspoon salt
Juice of ½ lemon
2 tbsp water
1 tbsp olive oil
1 thumb (5 cm) fresh ginger, peeled and cut into small sticks
1 teaspoon cumin seeds
½ teaspoon mustard seeds
1 red onion, sliced

STEPS FOR COOKING

1. First, mix all the ground spices and salt in a small bowl. Add the lemon juice and water.
2. Quickly stir in ginger and fry for a minute, then add cumin and mustard seeds. Let simmer for a minute and as soon as they start to sizzle and bud, add the onions and cauliflower florets. Fry for about 3-4 minutes - you want brown spots to appear on the cauliflower.
3. Pour the spice mixture over the cauliflower, stir well, then reduce the heat and put the lid on. Then let it steam for 8 minutes. Put in the tomato cubes, stir and cook for another 10-15 minutes, until the cauliflower is tender.

INGREDIENTS

1 medium-sized (approx. 800g) cauliflower, cut into small florets
2 tomatoes diced

STEPS FOR COOKING

Strawberry & Citrus Blend

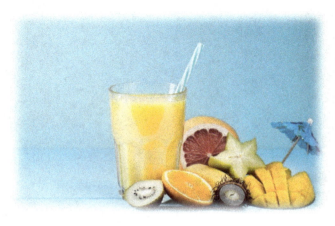

Time required: 35 minutes

Servings: 01

INGREDIENTS

75g (3oz) strawberries
1 apple, cored
1 orange, peeled
½ avocado, peeled and de-stoned
½ teaspoon matcha powder
Juice of 1 lime

STEPS FOR COOKING

1. Place all of the ingredients into a blender with enough water to cover them and process until smooth.

Raspberry and Blackcurrant Jelly

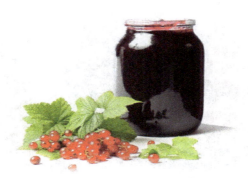

Time required: 3 hours

Servings: 02

INGREDIENTS

4 ounces raspberries (washed and dried)

2 leaves gelatin

4 ounces blackcurrants (washed and stalks removed)

2 tbsp granulated sugar

1¼ cups water (divided)

STEPS FOR COOKING

1. Divide the raspberries between 2 glasses.
2. Add the gelatin to a small bowl of cold water and allow to soften. Allow 1 cup of water per sheet.
3. Add the blackcurrants to a pan along with the sugar and ⅝ cup of water, and bring to a boil. Simmer vigorously for 5 minutes and remove the pan from the heat. Allow to stand for 2 minutes.
4. Squeeze any excess water out of the gelatin leaves and add them to the pan. Stir well until dissolved entirely. Stir in the remaining water.
5. Pour the liquid evenly into the 2 glasses, and place in the refrigerator to set for 3-8 hours.

Mince Stuffed Eggplants

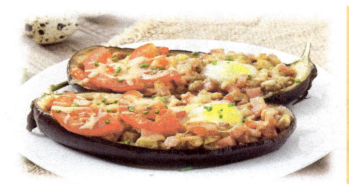

Time required: 85 minutes

Servings: 06

INGREDIENTS

4 oz. lean mince
6 large eggplants
1 egg
3 tbsp. dry red wine
½ cup cheddar, grated
Salt and pepper, to taste
1 red onion
2 tsp. olive oil
2 tbsp. tomato sauce
2 tbsp. parsley

STEPS FOR COOKING

1. Preheat oven to 350°F. Meanwhile, slice eggplants in 2 and scoop out the center part, leaving ½ inch of meat. Place eggplants in a microwavable dish with about ½" of water in the bottom.
2. Microwave on high for 4 minutes. In a saucepan, fry mince with onion for 5 minutes.
3. Add wine and let evaporate.
4. Add tomato sauce, salt, pepper, eggplant meat and cook for around 20 minutes until done.
5. Combine, mince sauce, cheese, egg, parsley, salt, and pepper in a large bowl and mix well. Pack firmly into eggplants.
6. Return eggplants to the dish you first microwaved them in and bake for 25 to 30 minutes, or until lightly browned on top.

Turkey Curry

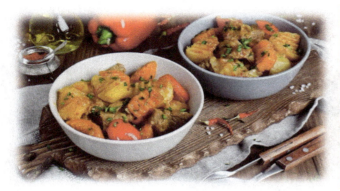

Time required: 45 minutes

Servings: 04

INGREDIENTS

450g (1lb) turkey breasts, chopped
100g (3½ oz) fresh rocket (arugula) leaves
5 cloves garlic, chopped
3 teaspoons medium curry powder
2 teaspoons turmeric powder
2 tablespoons fresh coriander (cilantro), finely chopped
2 bird's-eye chilies, chopped
2 red onions, chopped
400mls (14fl oz) full-fat coconut milk
2 tablespoons olive oil

STEPS FOR COOKING

1. Heat the olive oil in a saucepan, add the chopped red onions and cook them for around 5 minutes or until soft.
2. Stir in the garlic and the turkey and cook it for 7-8 minutes.
3. Stir in the turmeric, chilies and curry powder then add the coconut milk and coriander (cilantro).
4. Bring it to the boil, reduce the heat and simmer for around 10 minutes.
5. Scatter the rocket (arugula) onto plates and spoon the curry on top. Serve alongside brown rice.

Turkey Escalope with Sage, Trick and Parsley and Spiced Cauliflower 'Couscous'

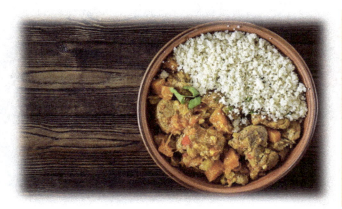

Time required: 25 minutes

Servings: 04

INGREDIENTS

5 oz. cauliflower, generally slashed
1 clove garlic, finely slashed
1.5 oz. red onion, finely hacked
1 10,000 foot stew, finely slashed
1tsp new ginger, finely hacked
2tbsp additional virgin olive oil
2tsp ground turmeric
1 oz. sun-dried tomatoes, finely cleaved
0.35 oz. parsley

STEPS FOR COOKING

1. Place the cauliflower in a food processor and heartbeat in 2-second blasts to finely slash it until it takes after couscous.
2. Put in a safe spot. Fry the garlic, red onion, stew and ginger in 1tsp of the oil until delicate however not shaded. Add the turmeric and cauliflower and cook for 1 moment.
3. Eliminate from the warmth and add the sun-dried tomatoes and a large portion of the parsley.
4. Coat the turkey escalope in the excess oil and sage at that point fry for 5-6 minutes, turning consistently.
5. At the point when cooked, add the lemon juice, remaining parsley, tricks

INGREDIENTS

5 oz. turkey escalope
1tsp dried sage
Juice 1/2 lemon
1tbsp escapades

STEPS FOR COOKING

and 1tbsp water to the skillet to make a sauce, at that point serve.

Baked Cod with Kale, Chicory and White Beans

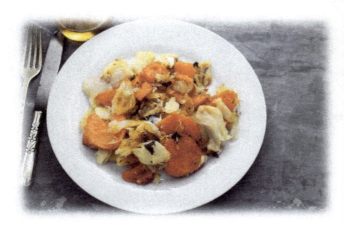

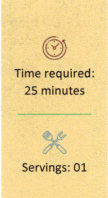

Time required: 25 minutes

Servings: 01

INGREDIENTS

150 g cod fillet
½ teaspoon extra-virgin olive oil
1 teaspoon chopped parsley
For the Beans:
50 g kale, sliced, the stems removed
1 teaspoon extra-virgin olive oil
30 g red onion
1 clove of garlic sliced
100 ml vegetable stock
75 g from the can or homemade white

STEPS FOR COOKING

1. Heat the oven to 200°C/gas. 6. Line the parchment paper with a small baking sheet. Steam or cook the kale until tender for 5–7 minutes, then set aside.

2. Rub the fish with parsley and olive oil and put on the prepared tray, and cook for 10 minutes in the oven. Meanwhile, over low to medium heat, heat the olive oil in a small saucepan and fry the red onion and garlic for 2-3 minutes until tender.

3. Attach the beans and stock and put them to a boil. Attach the chicory and cook for a few more minutes on low to medium heat. Take caution not to cook for too long. Using the mixture to stir the kale and eat with the tuna.

SHANNEN GALLOWEY
Sirtfood Diet Cookbook

INGREDIENTS

beans such as cannellini or haricot
1 head of chicory, halved lengthways and sliced

STEPS FOR COOKING

Chicken Fajitas

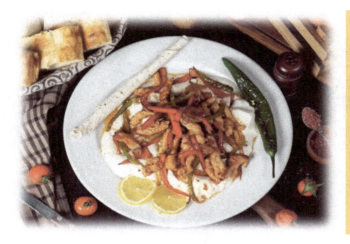

Time required: 25 minutes

Servings: 04

INGREDIENTS

2 chicken breast fillets
1 chilli pepper
1 clove of garlic
1 yellow pepper
1 green pepper
1 red onion
2 tablespoons oil
100 ml poultry broth
100 g corn kernels
salt
Cayenne pepper
2 tbsp chopped parsley
4 tortillas

STEPS FOR COOKING

1. Wash the chicken breasts and cut into small cubes. Wash and finely chop the chilli. Peel the garlic and press into the chilli. Wash, clean, core the peppers and cut into fine strips. Peel the onion, cut in half and also cut into strips.
2. Sweat the chicken cubes in hot oil, add the pepper strips and the onion and deglaze with the broth. Add the corn kernels, chilli and garlic and let everything simmer for 5-7 minutes at a low temperature.
3. Season to taste with salt and cayenne pepper, mix in 1 tablespoon of parsley and spread over the tortillas. Roll up and serve sprinkled with the rest of the parsley.

Green Tea Smoothie

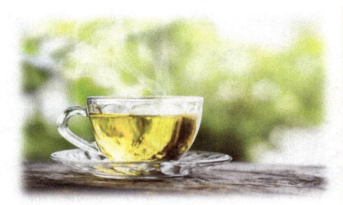

Time required: 5 minutes

Servings: 02

INGREDIENTS

2 ripe bananas (peeled)
1 cup milk
2 tsp Matcha green tea powder
½ tsp vanilla bean paste
6 ice cubes
2 tsp honey

STEPS FOR COOKING

1. In a food blender, combine the bananas, milk, Matcha green tea powder, vanilla bean paste, ice cubes, and honey.
2. Divide between 2 glasses and serve.

Turmeric Couscous with Edamame Beans

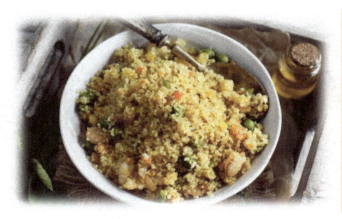

Time required: 25 minutes

Servings: 02

INGREDIENTS

½ yellow pepper, cubed
½ red pepper, cubed
1 tbsp. turmeric
½ cup red onion, finely sliced
¼ cup cherry tomatoes, chopped
2 tbsp. parsley, finely chopped
5 oz. couscous
2 tsp. extra virgin olive oil
½ eggplant
1 ½ edamame beans

STEPS FOR COOKING

1. Steam edamame for 5 minutes and set aside. Add 6 oz. salted boiling water to couscous and let rest until it absorbs the water.
2. In the meantime, heat a pan on medium-high heat.
3. Add oil, eggplant, peppers, onion and tomatoes, turmeric, salt, and pepper. Cook for 5 minutes on high heat.
4. Add the couscous and edamame.
5. Garnish with fresh parsley and serve.

Crude Brownie Bites

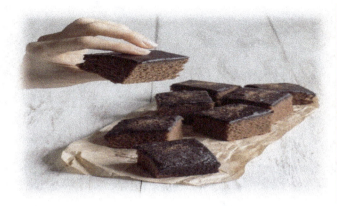

Time required: 5 minutes

Servings: 06

INGREDIENTS

2½ cups entire pecans
¼ cup almonds
2½ cups Medjool dates
1 cup cacao powder
1 teaspoon vanilla concentrate
⅛-¼ teaspoon ocean salt

STEPS FOR COOKING

1. Spot everything in a food processor until very much consolidated.
2. Fold into balls and spot on a heating sheet and freeze for 30 minutes or refrigerate for 2 hours.

Sirtfood Pizza

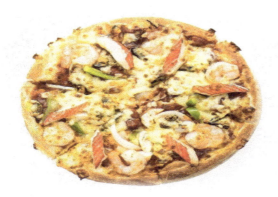

Time required: 40 minutes

Servings: 04

INGREDIENTS

For the Dough:
7g dry yeast
1 teaspoon brown sugar
300ml water
200g buckwheat flour
200g wheat flour for pasta
1 tablespoon of olive oil

For the Sauce:
1/2 red onion, finely chopped
1 clove of garlic, finely chopped
1 teaspoon of olive oil
1 teaspoon oregano, dried

STEPS FOR COOKING

For the Dough:
1. Dissolve dry yeast and sugar in water and leave covered for 15 minutes. Then mix the flours. Add the yeast water and oil and make a dough.
2. Preheat oven to 425 °. Then knead the dough well again and form two pizzas, each 30 cm in diameter, with a rolling pin on a floured work surface. Or you can form a thin pizza that fits on a whole baking sheet.
3. Spread the pizza dough on a baking tray lined with baking paper.

For the Sauce:
1. Fry the garlic, onion and sugar with olive oil, add the wine and oregano and cook briefly. Then add the tomatoes and cook on low heat for 30 minutes. Then set aside and add the fresh basil leaves.

SHANNEN GALLOWEY
Sirtfood Diet Cookbook

INGREDIENTS

2 tablespoons red wine
1 can of strained tomatoes (400ml)
1 pinch of brown sugar
5g basil leaves

STEPS FOR COOKING

2. Pizza topping and baking
3. Spread the desired amount of tomato sauce on the dough - leave the edges as free as possible, do not spread too thickly.
4. Then add the desired ingredients, for example sliced red onion and grilled eggplant
5. Goat cheese and cherry tomatoes
6. Chicken breast (grilled), red onions and olives Kale, chorizo and red onions
7. Then bake for about 12 minutes and, if desired, sprinkle with rocket, pepper and chili flakes.

Beef Burger with Sweet Potato Fries

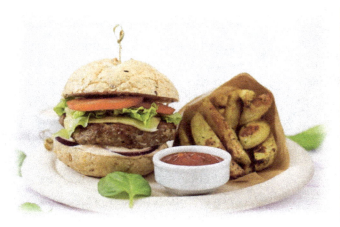

Time required: 45 minutes

Servings: 01

INGREDIENTS

125 g lean ground beef (5 percent fat)
15 g red onion, finely chopped
1 teaspoon finely chopped parsley
1 teaspoon extra-virgin olive oil

For the Fries:
150 g sweet potatoes
1 teaspoon extra-virgin olive oil
1 teaspoon dried rosemary
1 clove of garlic, unpeeled

For Serving:

STEPS FOR COOKING

1. Heat up to 220 ° C / gas in the oven. 7. Next, make the fries. Peel the sweet potato and cut it into French fries that are 1 cm thick. Mix them with the olive oil, the rosemary and the garlic cloves.

2. Place them on a baking sheet and cook until crispy, for 30 minutes. Mix the onion and parsley with the ground beef for the burger. When you have cookie cutters, you should use the largest cookie cutter in the package to shape your burger. Otherwise, to make a sound, even pie, use your hands.

3. Heat a pan over medium heat, add the olive oil and put on one side of the pan the burger and on the other the onion rings. Cook the burger on each

SHANNEN GALLOWEY
Sirtfood Diet Cookbook

INGREDIENTS

10 g cheddar cheese, sliced or grated
150 g red onion, cut into rings
30 g tomato, cut
10 g rocket
1 pickle (optional)

STEPS FOR COOKING

side for 6 minutes, ensuring that it is cooked. To taste, cook the onion rings.

4. Pour the cheese and red onion on top when the burger is grilled and put them for a minute in the hot oven to melt the cheese.
5. Take out the tomatoes, rocket and pickles and place on top. Serve with the fries.

Yellow Lentil Soup with Chilli, Ginger and Turmeric

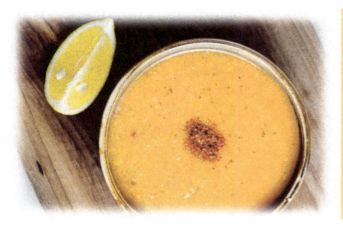

Time required: 45 minutes

Servings: 04

INGREDIENTS

200 g organic yellow lentils
200 ml coconut milk
1 teaspoon Thai red curry paste
500 ml vegetable stock, homemade
2 shallots
2 cloves of garlic
1 chilli pepper, raw
8 stalks of coriander, fresh
2 stalks of celery, raw
10 g ginger
1 lime organic quality

STEPS FOR COOKING

1. Peel and finely dice shallots. Skin the garlic and cut into fine slices. Wash and dry celery and cut into thin slices.
2. Let the coconut oil get hot in a high pot and fry the celery in it for about 5 minutes at a medium temperature, so it will be pleasantly soft.
3. Then add the curry paste and fry it, add the shallots and garlic and sweat everything until translucent.
4. Pour a little vegetable stock on top. Now put the lentils in the pot and cook for 10 minutes, gradually adding the vegetable stock.
5. Slice the ginger and add to the soup. Let everything cook at a low

INGREDIENTS

1 teaspoon turmeric powder
1/2 teaspoon curry powder
1 teaspoon five spices powder
1/2 teaspoon cumin
1-star anise
1 teaspoon sea salt (fleur de sel)
1 pinch of black pepper
2 tbsp coconut oil
Drinking water as needed

STEPS FOR COOKING

temperature for about 20 minutes, stirring occasionally.

6. To make the soup a little thicker, briefly add the hand blender 2-3 times and purée the soup gently. Wash the lime warm, use the grater to grate the zest into small zest and stir into the soup.

7. Rinse the chilli pepper and cut into fine rings. Wash off the coriander and peel off the leaves. Season the soup with salt and pepper, garnish with the coriander and the chilli pepper and serve.

Turmeric Tea

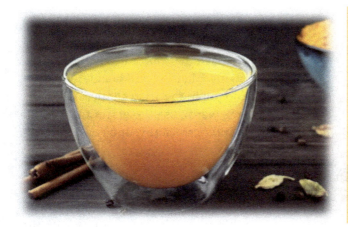

Time required: 5 minutes

Servings: 02

INGREDIENTS

2 cups water
3 tsp ground turmeric
1 tbsp fresh ginger (peeled and grated)
Zest of 1 small orange
Honey (to serve)

STEPS FOR COOKING

1. Bring 2 cups of water to boil.
2. Add the ground turmeric, grated ginger, and orange zest to a jug or teapot. Pour the boiling water over the mixture in the jug and infuse for 5 minutes. Strain the tea through a sieve into 2 cups.
3. Add a slice of lemon and sweeten to taste with honey.

Potato Salad

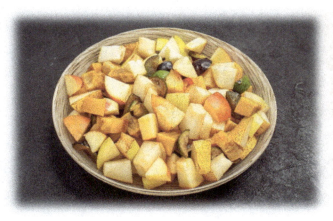

Time required: 25 minutes

Servings: 02

INGREDIENTS

7 oz. celery, generally slashed
3.5 oz. apple, generally slashed
1.77 oz. pecans, generally slashed
1 little red onion, generally cleaved
1 head of chicory, hacked
0.35 oz. level parsley, hacked
1 tbsp tricks
0.35 oz. lovage or celery leaves, generally hacked
For the Dressing:
1 tbsp additional virgin olive oil

STEPS FOR COOKING

1. Blend the celery, apple, pecans, onion, parsley, tricks and lovage/celery in a medium-sized plate of mixed greens bowl and blend.
2. Make the dressing by whisking together the oil, vinegar, mustard and lemon juice. Drizzle over the plate of mixed greens, blend and serve!

INGREDIENTS

1 tsp balsamic vinegar
1 teaspoon Dijon mustard
Juice of a large portion of a lemon

STEPS FOR COOKING

Black Bean Salsa

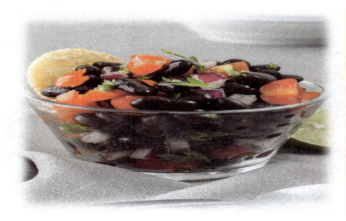

Time required: 10 minutes

Servings: 04

INGREDIENTS

1 tablespoon coconut aminos
½ teaspoon cumin, ground
1 cup canned black beans, no salt
1 cup salsa
6 cups romaine lettuce, torn
½ cup avocado, peeled, pitted and cubed

STEPS FOR COOKING

1. Take a bowl and add beans, alongside other ingredients. Toss well and serve.
2. Enjoy!

Kale and Butternut Bowls

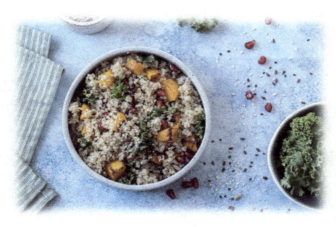

Time required: 60 minutes

Servings: 04

INGREDIENTS

1 Red onion, diced
1 Butternut squash, seeds removed and cut into quarters
3 cups Kale, chopped
2 Garlic, minced
1 tablespoon Extra virgin olive oil
1 teaspoon Oregano
.25 teaspoon Cinnamon
.5 teaspoon Turmeric powder
1 teaspoon Sea salt
1 Avocado, sliced
4 Eggs
.25 cup Parsley, chopped -
.25 teaspoon Black pepper, ground

STEPS FOR COOKING

1. Set the oven at four hundred- and twenty-degrees Fahrenheit. Place the butternut squash upside down on a pan so that the side of the skin faces upward. Roast the butternut squash for about twenty-five to thirty minutes, until the pork is tender.

2. Enable the butternut squash to cool down enough to be easy to touch, and then peel your hands off the flesh. Break the butternut squash into bite-size cubes.

3. Heat the extra virgin olive oil over a moderate medium - high heat skillet and sauté the onion for about five minutes until it is translucent. Connect the kale, garlic, and seasonings and simmer until the kale wilts. In the butternut squash, add.

SHANNEN GALLOWEY
Sirtfood Diet Cookbook

INGREDIENTS	STEPS FOR COOKING
	4. Divide the skillet mixture into four serving bowls and finish each with your favorite fried egg, sliced avocado, and parsley.

Sweet Potato Soup

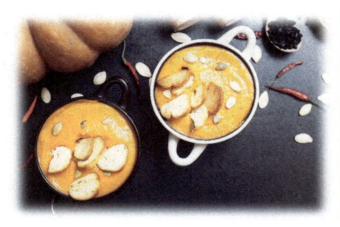

Time required: 45 minutes

Servings: 04

INGREDIENTS

1 red onion
1 clove of garlic
2 carrots
400 g sweet potatoes
150 g celeriac (1 piece)
2 tbsp olive oil
Iodized salt with fluoride Chilli powder
1 l vegetable stock
200 g kale
40 g peanuts
200 g yogurt

STEPS FOR COOKING

1. Skin, peel and peel the onion, garlic, carrots, sweet potatoes and celery and cut into small cubes.
2. Put the oil in a saucepan, let it get hot and sear the diced vegetables in it at a high temperature for 3 minutes. Refine with salt and chilli powder, pour the stock into the saucepan and let it simmer for about 20 minutes at a low temperature.
3. In the meantime, clean the kale thoroughly, remove it from the hard stalks and blanch the leaves in boiling salted water for 1-2 minutes. Pour off the kale, rinse with cold water, wring out and then roughly chop.
4. Melt the butter in a pan and let it get hot. Sweat the kale in it over a

INGREDIENTS	STEPS FOR COOKING
	medium heat for about 5 minutes. Meanwhile, chop peanuts. 5. Puree the soup to a homogeneous mass and remove from the heat. Stir 120 g of yogurt into the soup. Refine with salt and chili powder. 6. Divide the sweet potato soup into 4 deep plates and garnish a yogurt topping with the rest of the yogurt. Distribute the kale and nuts decoratively on the soup and serve.

Easy Shrimp Salad

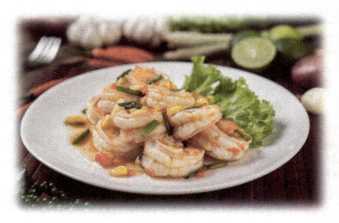

Time required: 5 minutes

Servings: 02

INGREDIENTS

2 cups red endive, finely sliced
1 cup cherry tomatoes, halved
1 tsp. of extra virgin olive oil
1 tbsp. parsley, chopped
3 oz. celery, sliced
6 walnuts, chopped
2 oz. red onion-sliced
1 cup yellow pepper, cubed
½ lemon, juiced
6 oz. steamed shrimps

STEPS FOR COOKING

1. Put red endive on a large plate. Evenly distribute on top finely sliced onion, yellow pepper, cherry tomatoes walnuts, celery, and parsley.
2. Mix oil, lemon juice with a pinch of salt and pepper and distribute the dressing on top.

New Saag Paneer

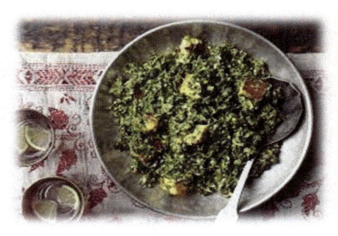

Time required: 25 minutes

Servings: 02

INGREDIENTS

2 tsp rapeseed oil
7 oz. paneer. cut into shapes
Salt and newly ground dark pepper
1 red onion, cleaved
1 little thumb (3 cm) new ginger, stripped and cut into matchsticks
1 clove garlic, stripped and daintily cut
1 green stew, deseeded and finely cut
3.5 oz. cherry tomatoes, split
1/2 tsp ground coriander

STEPS FOR COOKING

1. Heat the oil in a wide lidded griddle over a high warmth. Season the paneer liberally with salt and pepper and throw into the skillet. Fry for a couple of moments until brilliant, mixing regularly. Eliminate from the container with an opened spoon and put in a safe spot.

2. Reduce the warmth and add the onion. Fry for 5 minutes prior to adding the ginger, garlic and bean stew. Cook for another couple of minutes prior to adding the cherry tomatoes. Put the top on the skillet and cook for a further 5 minutes.

3. Add the flavors and salt, at that point mix. Return the paneer to the container and mix until covered. Add the spinach to the container along

INGREDIENTS

1/2 tsp ground cumin
1/2 tsp ground turmeric
1/2 tsp gentle bean stew powder
1/2 tsp salt
3.5 oz. new spinach leaves
Little small bunch (0.35 oz.) parsley, slashed Little small bunch (0.35 oz.) coriander, slashed

STEPS FOR COOKING

with the parsley and coriander and put the cover on. Permit the spinach to shrink for 1-2 minutes, at that point consolidate into the dish. Serve right away.

Corn Spread

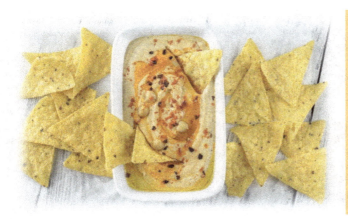

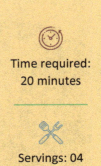

Time required: 20 minutes

Servings: 04

INGREDIENTS

1 medium zucchini
1 tablespoon grated red onion
2 extra-large eggs lightly beaten
3 tablespoons all-purpose flour
½ tablespoons ground black pepper
½ tablespoon salt
vegetable oil
1 teaspoon of baking powder

STEPS FOR COOKING

1. Preheat the oven to over 300 degrees Fahrenheit.
2. In a mixing bowl, grate the zucchini and add the onions and eggs right away.
3. Combine the flour, baking powder, salt, and pepper in a mixing bowl.
4. Add the vegetable oil to a big sauté pan and steam over medium heat.
5. Reduce the heat to medium-low and pour the batter into the pan once the oil is hot. Cook both sides for about 2 minutes.

Moroccan Leeks Snack

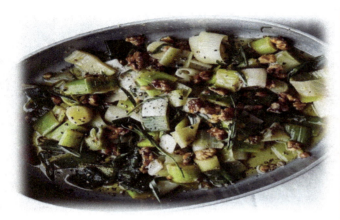

Time required: 10 minutes

Servings: 04

INGREDIENTS

1 bunch radish, sliced 3 cups leeks, chopped
1 ½ cups olives, pitted and sliced
Pinch turmeric powder
2 tablespoons essential olive oil
1 cup cilantro, chopped

STEPS FOR COOKING

1. Take a bowl and mix in radishes, leeks, olives and cilantro. Mix well.
2. Season with pepper, oil, turmeric and toss well. Serve and enjoy!

Best Ever Bran Muffins

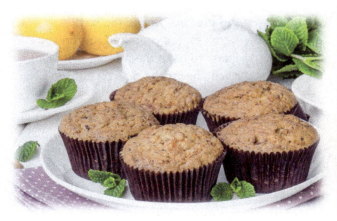

Time required: 25 minutes

Servings: 12

INGREDIENTS

.75 cup Whole-wheat flour -
1 cup All-purpose flour
2.25 cups All-Bran Cereal
.5 cup Date sugar
.5 teaspoon Sea salt
2 teaspoons Baking powder
1.75 cup Soy yogurt, plain
2 Eggs
.33 cup Extra virgin olive oil
.25 cup Molasses
2 teaspoons Vanilla extract
.5 cup Dried raisins, cherries, or currants

STEPS FOR COOKING

1. Prepare a muffin pan with paper liners as the oven preheats to four-hundred degrees Fahrenheit.
2. Along with the dried fruit, pour half of the All-Bran cereal into a food processor or blender. Pulse the mixture until it is finely chopped and when done, move it to a dish. The remaining All-Bran, both flours, sea salt, baking soda, and date sugar, are added to the dish. Please give it a nice blend and set the bowl aside.
3. Whisk the soy yogurt, eggs, extra virgin olive oil, molasses, and vanilla together in another dish. Stir this mixture into the mixture of cereal flour, taking care, not to over blend.
4. For up to two weeks, cool the batter in the refrigerator or instantly bake

INGREDIENTS	STEPS FOR COOKING
	the muffins. Divide the batter between the prepared muffin cup liners to bake the muffin, just filling each liner three-quarters of the way up.
5. Bake the muffins until they are cleanly removed with an inserted toothpick, and when they spring back when struck. It should take 15 to 18 minutes.

Stew with Green Vegetables

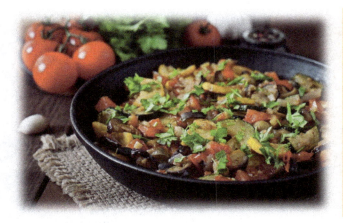

Time required: 60 minutes

Servings: 04

INGREDIENTS

3 red onions
2 cloves of garlic
100 g soft chorizo
300 g potatoes (5 potatoes)
4 tbsp olive oil
1 pinch of cumin
800 ml classic vegetable stock
450 g kale
1/2 organic lemon
3 pickled piri piri
350 g prawns (ready to cook; without head and shell)
Salt pepper

STEPS FOR COOKING

1. Peel the onions and garlic and dice them very finely. Cut the sausage into fine cubes. Remove the potatoes from the skin, wash and also dice. Melt 2 tablespoons of olive oil in a saucepan. Sweat the onions in it until translucent for 7-8 minutes and stir occasionally.

2. Add the garlic and chorizo to the pan and fry everything together for another 2 minutes.

3. Now add the cumin, potatoes and stock, bring to the boil once, then reduce the heat and simmer over medium heat for about 20 minutes.

4. In the meantime, clean the kale, wash it thoroughly and wring it out well. Cut the kale into very fine strips or pull apart.

INGREDIENTS	STEPS FOR COOKING
	5. Wash the lemon with hot water, pat dry and cut some zest into zest. Pat the piri pods dry, taking care not to throw away the oil. Chop the pods very finely and mix with the remaining oil and lemon zest.
	6. Use a hand blender to puree the potatoes, onions, garlic and sausage in the broth to make a homogeneous soup. Let the kale slide into the stock and boil everything down for another 10 minutes over medium heat.
	7. Wash the shrimp thoroughly, pat dry and add to the stew. Bring everything to the boil again, reduce the heat again and let it simmer for another 2 minutes. Refine with salt and pepper. Drizzle the stew with the piri piri oil decoratively and serve in the plates.

Tuscan Bean Stew

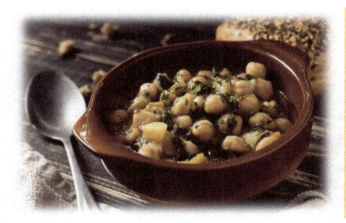

Time required: 45 minutes

Servings: 01

INGREDIENTS

1 tbsp extra-virgin olive oil
1¾ ounces red onion (peeled and finely chopped)
1 ounce carrot (peeled and finely chopped)
1 ounce celery (trimmed and chopped)
1 clove garlic (peeled and chopped)
½ bird's eye chili (finely chopped)
1 tsp Herbes de Provence
⅗ cup vegetable stock

STEPS FOR COOKING

1. Add the oil to a pan, and over low to moderate heat, fry the onion, carrots, celery, chili, and Herbes de Provence, until the onion is softened but not colored.
2. Pour in the stock and add the tomatoes, tomato puree and bring to a boil. Add the mixed beans, and simmer for 30 minutes.
3. Add the kale and cook for an additional 5-10 minutes, until tender. Stir in the parsley.
4. In the meantime, cook the buckwheat according to the package directions. Drain the buckwheat and serve with the stew.

INGREDIENTS

1 (14-ounce) chopped Italian tomatoes
1 tsp tomato purée
7 ounces canned mixed beans
1¾ ounces kale (coarsely chopped)
1 tbsp fresh parsley (coarsely chopped)
1½ ounces buckwheat

STEPS FOR COOKING

Chicken Breakfast Skillet

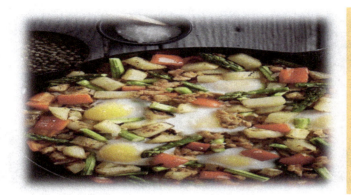

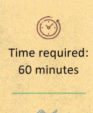

Time required: 60 minutes

Servings: 02

INGREDIENTS

1 chicken breast
3 ounces ground sausage
2 eggs
3 slices bacon
½ teaspoon garlic powder
½ teaspoon ground black pepper

STEPS FOR COOKING

1. Chop the bacon and chicken breast into pieces roughly one inch in size. Add the bacon to a skillet over medium heat and cook for two minutes, stirring frequently. Once the bacon grease has begun to accumulate in the pan, stir in the diced chicken and ground or crumbled sausage.

2. Add garlic powder and pepper to the meat in the skillet. Brown the meat over medium-high heat for about six to eight minutes.

3. Reduce heat to medium. On opposite sides of the pan, clear two pockets of space for the eggs. Crack the eggs into the skillet and break the yolks apart. Cover the skillet and allow cooking so that the egg whites are firm about 10 minutes. Uncover and scoop onto a plate to serve.

Green Shakshuka

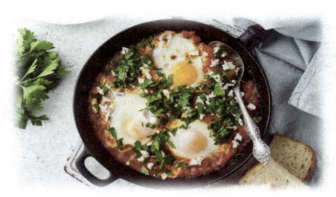

Time required: 25 minutes

Servings: 03

INGREDIENTS

1 Zucchini, grated
9 ounces Brussels sprouts, finely sliced or shaved
1 Red onion, diced
2 tablespoons Olive oil
5 Eggs
.25 cup, Parsley chopped
2 cups Kale chopped
.5 teaspoon Sea salt
1 teaspoon Cumin
1 Avocado, sliced

STEPS FOR COOKING

1. Sauté the red onion in the olive oil in a wide steel skillet for about three minutes before it becomes partially translucent. Add in the minced garlic and cook the mixture of onion/garlic for an extra minute.
2. In the skillet containing the onion and garlic, add the Brussels sprouts and roast for four to five minutes until softened, stirring regularly. Stir in the spices and zucchini, then simmer for an extra minute.
3. Stir in the skillet with the kale and continue stirring until it starts to wilt. Lower the heat to a low level.
4. The shakshuka mixture in the skillet is flattened with a spatula, and five small wells are formed for the eggs to come in. In each of the shakshuka wells, crack an egg and cover the

INGREDIENTS

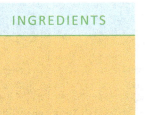

STEPS FOR COOKING

skillet with a lid to steam the eggs until they fit your taste.

5. Round the dish off with the avocado and parsley, and serve immediately.

Buckwheat Superfood Muesli

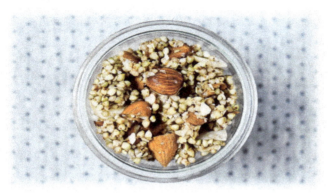

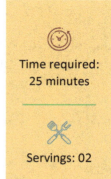

Time required: 25 minutes

Servings: 02

INGREDIENTS

0.7 oz. buckwheat pieces
0.35 oz. buckwheat puffs
10.2 oz. coconut pieces or dried up coconut
1.5 oz. Medjool dates, hollowed and cleaved
10.2 oz. pecans, cleaved
0.35 oz. cocoa nibs
3.5 oz. strawberries, hulled and cleaved
3.5 oz. plain Greek yogurt (or veggie lover elective, for example, soy or coconut yogurt)

STEPS FOR COOKING

1. Blend the entirety of the above Ingredients together (leave out the strawberries and yogurt if not serving straight away).
2. On the off chance that you need to make this in mass or set it up the prior night, essentially join the dry Ingredients and store it in an impenetrable compartment.
3. All you require to do the following day is add the strawberries and yogurt and it's all set.

Pineapple & Cucumber Smoothie

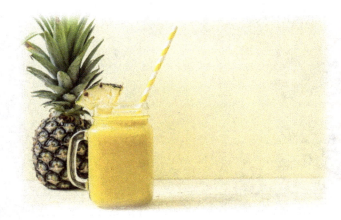

Time required: 5 minutes

Servings: 01

INGREDIENTS

50g (2oz) cucumber
1 stalk of celery
2 slices of fresh pineapple
2 sprigs of parsley
½ teaspoon matcha powder
Squeeze of lemon juice

STEPS FOR COOKING

1. Place all of the ingredients into blender with enough water to cover them and blitz until smooth.

Roasted Cajun Nuts

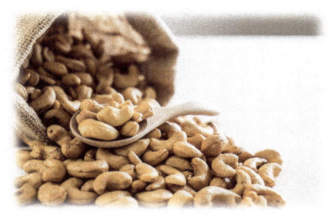

Time required: 30 minutes

Servings: 02

INGREDIENTS

250 g blanched peanuts or a mixture of pecans, walnuts and hazelnuts
1 tbsp extra-virgin olive oil or coconut oil
1 teaspoon paprika
1 teaspoon dried thyme
1 teaspoon sea salt
1 teaspoon oregano
1 teaspoon chili powder

STEPS FOR COOKING

1. Heat the oven to a temperature of 160°C.
2. Mix and blend all the ingredients with the nuts and oil. On a roasting pan, put the nuts in a single layer and sauté them for 25-30 minutes.
3. In a cup, placed the roasted nuts. Store in an airtight jar for up to two days after cooling completely.

Frozen Chocolate Grapes

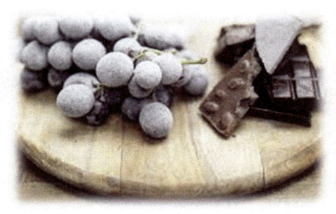

Time required: 15 minutes

Servings: 04

INGREDIENTS

50 g 70% dark chocolate
150 g red seedless grapes

STEPS FOR COOKING

1. Line a baking sheet with a sheet of silicone or parchment paper.
2. Chop the chocolate into small pieces and place in a small heat-resistant bowl. Slightly heat a small pan with water and place the bowl with the chocolate on it.
3. Heat and stir the chocolate so it melts slowly and remove it from the heat if there are any lumps left. Keep stirring the chocolate until it is completely melted (this will help avoid white spots or blooming on the chocolate).
4. Dip the grapes one after the other in the chocolate so that they are half covered and immediately place on the baking sheet. Continue with all the grapes. Let the chocolate harden at room temperature before putting it in the freezer. After freezing, the grapes

INGREDIENTS

STEPS FOR COOKING

can be transferred to a suitable freezer container.

5. Serve or add in portions of 10-12 grapes at once and save a few if necessary.

Choc Chip Granola

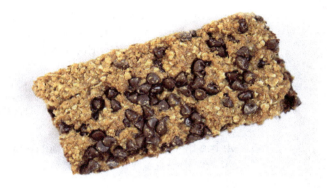

Time required: 35 minutes

Servings: 08

INGREDIENTS

7 ounces jumbo oats
1¾ ounces pecans (coarsely chopped)
2 tbsp light olive oil
¾ ounce butter
1 tbsp dark brown sugar 2 tbsp pure maple syrup
2 ounces good-quality 85% cocoa dark chocolate chips

STEPS FOR COOKING

1. Preheat the main oven to 320 degrees F. Using baking parchment, line a baking tray.
2. In a bowl, combine the oats with the pecans.
3. Heat the oil in a small pan, and add the butter, brown sugar, and maple syrup. Cook until the butter has melted and the sugar and maple syrup dissolved. Do not allow the mixture to boil.
4. Pour the syrup over the oat mixture and stir well until the oats are entirely covered.
5. Distribute the granola over the prepared baking tray, spreading it into the corners of the baking tray. Instead of spreading evenly, leave clumps of the granola with spacing.

INGREDIENTS	STEPS FOR COOKING
	6. Bake the granola in the oven for 20 minutes until the edges are golden. Take the granola out of the oven and allow to cool while on the tray.
7. When completely cool, using your fingers, break up any of the larger clumps
8. on the baking tray and mix in the dark chocolate chips.
9. Transfer the granola to an airtight resealable jar and store for up to 14 days.

Walnut Butter

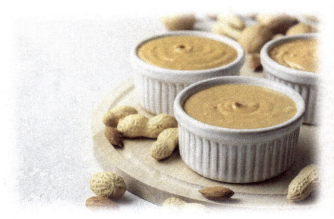

Time required: 45 minutes

Servings: 02

INGREDIENTS

350 g walnuts
2 teaspoons of extra-virgin olive oil
1 tsp water

STEPS FOR COOKING

1. In a food processor, put the walnuts and blend for around 2 minutes until you have fine crumbs.
2. Add the oil and water steadily and proceed until you have a smooth butter. If packed in an airtight jar in your freezer, it can be stored for up to 1 week.

Chocolate Dessert with Dates and Walnuts

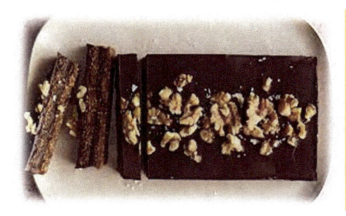

Time required: 25 minutes

Servings: 02

INGREDIENTS

4 Medjool dates, pitted
2 tbsp. cocoa powder
1 cup milk, skimmed
1 tsp. agar powder
1 tbsp. peanut butter
1 pinch of salt
½ tsp. cinnamon
2 walnuts
1 tsp. whole wheat flour

STEPS FOR COOKING

1. Blitz dates, peanut butter, and 1tbsp. milk in a food processor.
2. Put the mix in a pan; add cocoa, cinnamon, salt, flour, agar powder.
3. Add the remaining hot milk bit by bit and mix well to obtain a smooth mixture.
4. Turn the heat on, bring to a boil and cook around 6-8 minutes until dense.
5. Divide into 2 cups, let cool, and put in the fridge.
6. Add chopped walnuts before serving.

Blueberry Smoothie

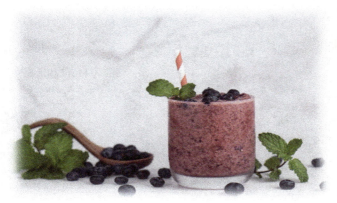

Time required: 5 minutes

Servings: 02

INGREDIENTS

1 ready banana
3.5 oz. blueberries
3.5 oz. blackberries
2 tbsp normal yogurt 200ml milk

STEPS FOR COOKING

1. Mix all the Ingredients together until smooth.

Avocado, Celery & Pineapple Smoothie

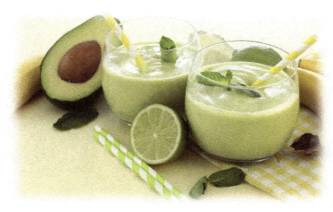

Time required: 5 minutes

Servings: 04

INGREDIENTS

50g (2oz) fresh pineapple, peeled and chopped
3 stalks of celery
1 avocado, peeled & de-stoned
1 tsp fresh parsley
½ tsp matcha powder Juice of ½ lemon

STEPS FOR COOKING

1. Place all of the ingredients into a blender and add enough water to cover them.
2. Process until creamy and smooth.

Sirtfood Bites

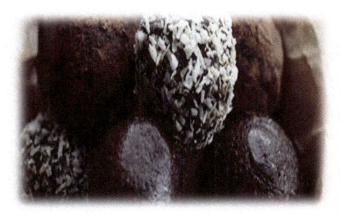

Time required: 25 minutes

Servings: 12

INGREDIENTS

120 g walnuts
30 g dark chocolate (85 percent cocoa solids), broken into pieces or cocoa nibs
250 g Medjool dates, pitted
1 tbsp cocoa powder (100 percent)
1 tbsp ground turmeric
1 tbsp extra-virgin olive oil
1 vanilla pod or 1 teaspoon vanilla extract
1–2 tbsp water (optional)

STEPS FOR COOKING

1. In a food processor, put the walnuts and chocolate and mix until you have a fine powder. Apply all the other ingredients except the water and combine until a ball shapes the mixture. If the mixture is dry, you should add water, but be careful - you do not want it to be too wet.

2. Shape the mixture with your hands into bite-sized balls and refrigerate for at least 1 hour before consuming it in an airtight dish.

3. For a different outcome, if you would like, roll any of the balls in more cocoa powder or dried coconut. The canapes can be kept for up to a week in the refrigerator.

CPSIA information can be obtained
at www.ICGtesting.com
Printed in the USA
BVHW091116240521
607998BV00011B/1645